AF686819

A DIRTY LITTLE *Secret*

THE STORY OF RICHARD, A VICTIM OF FETAL ALCOHOL SYNDROME

SHERRY T. FORD

Copyright © 2026 Sherry T. Ford.

All rights reserved. No part of this book may be reproduced, stored, or transmitted by any means—whether auditory, graphic, mechanical, or electronic—without written permission of both publisher and author, except in the case of brief excerpts used in critical articles and reviews. Unauthorized reproduction of any part of this work is illegal and is punishable by law.

ISBN: 979-8-90301-085-1 (sc)
ISBN: 979-8-90301-086-8 (hc)
ISBN: 979-8-90301-087-5 (e)

Because of the dynamic nature of the Internet, any web addresses or links contained in this book may have changed since publication and may no longer be valid. The views expressed in this work are solely those of the author and do not necessarily reflect the views of the publisher, and the publisher hereby disclaims any responsibility for them.

THE EWINGS PUBLISHING

One Galleria Blvd., Suite 1900, Metairie, LA 70001
(504) 702-6708

In loving memory of my brother,
Steven, who endured more than his share.

CONTENTS

INTRODUCTION

This memoir is a true story about the very short and tragic life of my nephew, Richard. Sadly, Richard's mother consumed alcohol during her pregnancy, and as a result of this prenatal exposure to alcohol, he sustained irreversible, life-challenging deficits, which ultimately lead to his death, and that of another. These deficits included poor judgment, insight, and social skills, oppositional behavior, and difficulty in learning. Unfortunately, his shortcomings were not easily recognizable to those who did not know him well. In fact, Richard appeared quite normal to most who knew and worked with him for short periods of time. Educators, for example, believed he was a sweet adolescent and budding young man with some emotional and attention deficit problems. But those of us who knew him very well feared for his future and his ability to make his way in the world safely.

This is a story that must be written because every day children are born with some degree of prenatal, alcohol-induced brain damage. This damage is permanent and totally preventable. It may not be initially visible, but as the child develops the deficits in judgment, awareness and behavior become increasingly more apparent. One might ask, "Why is this happening?" Certainly in a world where the facts are widely known by professionals you would expect people to have an awareness and understanding of the consequences of drinking during pregnancy. But far too many people do not understand the consequences of prenatal drinking.

For reasons I do not fully understand, public education about ***Fetal Alcohol Spectrum Disorders*** (FASD), or ***Fetal Alcohol Syndrome*** (FAS) is inadequate, and possibly why the condition remains under-diagnosed. The link between prenatal alcohol use and brain damage has been noted during the earliest of times, dating back to the Bible. Yet false claims that tout the safety of modest alcohol consumption during pregnancy continue to circulate among our society promoting a false sense of safety for this behavior. One day I decided to make random visits to six OB-GYN practices in my hometown of Baltimore, Maryland and not one office had brochures sitting out, or posters hanging, about the risks of prenatal alcohol consumption. There is no excuse for this since the Center for Disease Control (CDC) offers brochures and posters free of charge!

Embarrassingly, even I must admit as a nurse, that I was unaware of the full consequences of prenatal drinking until I took over the care of my nephew. The fact that alcohol is a teratogen (neurotoxin) that can interfere with human development at any stage of a pregnancy and cause damage to the fetus, was not stressed in my professional training. As a result, I was left believing the myth that drinking a small amount of alcohol during pregnancy is acceptable, safe behavior. Despite the overwhelming amount of FASD facts documented in medical journals, the commendable efforts of the National Organization on Fetal Alcohol Syndrome (NOFAS) to educate the public, the CDC's wealth of information available at no cost and easily downloaded from their website, and the Surgeon General's Advisory Report, knowledge about the full impact and danger of prenatal alcohol exposure continues to escape much of the population.

It is my hope that this memoir makes a difference. I challenge all who read it to spread the word, but I warn my readers that pregnant women who like to drink do not appreciate being told to stop. This I know from personal experience! But do not let this hinder you because a child's well-being is at stake. Print out the *Surgeon General's Advisory on Alcohol Use in Pregnancy* and pass it along to your pregnant friends and relatives. Refer them to the NOFAS website (www.nofas.org) for the facts. Ask your doctors (obstetricians, gynecologists, primary physicians, etc.) to download (or order) and display the free posters and pamphlets that NOFAS and the CDC offer (or do it yourself and deliver the information to them). Help to promote the facts and stop the dirty little secret!

Our children are our most valuable resource.
To limit their potential, before they are born,
is a crime of immeasurable magnitude.

CHAPTER 1

HUSBAND AND WIVES

My brother Steven was a loving and caring person. He was also extremely intelligent and independent, able to succeed first as a pharmacist, and then later as an accountant. Yet he lacked a key attribute for complete success; self-esteem. Growing up he struggled with insecurity and self-consciousness, labeled by some as an introvert. His short stature and large nose contributed to his poor self-image, and as he entered adulthood his over-eating, and subsequent obesity, further perpetuated his negative self-view.

As you might have guessed, Steven was not especially popular with women. He was definitely handsome, but extremely quiet and withdrawn in their company, always fearful of rejection. A blind date with a woman, who exhibited similar self-esteem issues as himself, turned into a co-dependent relationship, ultimately leading to marriage. The marriage lasted 10 years, and although a daughter was born, there was not enough love to sustain the union. After the divorce, Steven was not in a hurry to seek out another partner. So he lived alone as he approached the age of 40, suffered with depression, and ate more.

Fighting loneliness, Steven decided to join a bowling league. Bowling, along with playing cards and golf, had long been one of his passions, and it was here that he met his second wife. His second wife was not like him at all. She was very attractive and self-confident, outgoing and affectionate, athletic and fit, and accepting of everyone. Five years his junior and never married, she took to my brother immediately. I think Steven was in shock over all the love and attention she gave him. Never in his life had he experienced such strong affection and acceptance. Within a few months they announced their engagement.

I don't know how long it took for Steven to discover his new wife's addiction, but I feel certain it was within their first year of marriage. That addiction was alcoholism. I suspected the problem within a few months of their marriage, but hoped it was not as bad as I thought. In retrospect, I can see how powerful denial can be. I wanted my brother to be happy, and his new wife seemed to be the ticket. Their marriage seemed strong, filled with love and compatibility. It seemed like a marriage made in heaven; she overlooked his over-eating/obesity, and he overlooked her excessive drinking/alcoholism.

A year later the couple bought a home, and shortly thereafter (1987) their first son, Richard, was born. Richard was an active child; "all boy" people would say. He went from one activity to another, always moving on to something else. I guess you could say he ran circles around all of us. He just seemed like a normal, a little hyper, child. But his mother rarely seemed normal now. Her drinking was out of control. Steven tried to cover for her, but it was becoming increasingly difficult given her frequent slurred speech and unsteady gait. Then came the news of another pregnancy and Steven knew she needed help. With the help of family he convinced her of the need for inpatient alcohol rehabilitation. This was the saving grace for his second son born in 1989, a tiny, but healthy baby boy.

Despite all treatment efforts, his wife could not remain sober. In addition, she began seeking relationships outside the marriage. In the year 1991 Steven finally reached his limit, although he never stopped loving his second wife. He asked her to leave, and he sought and received legal custody of both his sons. She did not put up a fight.

CHAPTER 2

SELF DESTRUCTION BY ALCOHOL

Steven's wife moved out without a fight. She had a boyfriend who was ready and willing to take her in, and she was amenable to having supervised visitation with her sons. Her visits were few, and her struggle with alcoholism became a losing battle.

Several months passed, and then one morning Steven heard an unexpected knock at his door. He opened it to find a very sickly looking wife. He later told me in detail how shockingly ill she appeared. Disheveled in appearance, jaundiced and thin, and reeking of alcohol, she asked him for help. She asked if he would take care of her until she could "get back on her feet." With no questions asked, he told her he would do his best to help, but he expressed concern over her current condition and insisted on taking her to the hospital for evaluation first. She agreed to go, and he escorted her to the car. After asking a neighbor to watch the boys, Steven began his drive to the closest hospital emergency room.

The hospital was just five miles from his home, yet Steven was worried she would pass out next to him. He kept glancing at her in disbelief over how weak, debilitated and intoxicated she appeared. Her eyes were now closed, she was filled with congestion, and her coughing was persistent. As he pulled into the emergency parking area he thought she had fallen asleep. But when he tried to arouse her she was unresponsive. Steven then left her and ran to the emergency room entrance yelling for help. He screamed, "please come help my wife, I think she fainted in the car."

An emergency team responded quickly and followed my brother to his car, but to their dismay they determined that his wife had suffered an alcohol-induced cardiac arrest. Rescue efforts were initiated, however, there was severe oxygen deprivation to her brain. Her heart rate was restored, but she remained in a comatose state. She was admitted to the hospital and treated for several weeks with no progress noted in her condition. Then she was transferred to a nursing and rehabilitation center where she received maintenance care.

After several years, sometime around the year 2000, Steven's wife regained consciousness, however, she remained severely cognitively impaired and bedridden. She was unable to move her limbs and therefore could not walk or feed herself. Her language and comprehension ability was poor, and it was doubtful that she could recognize her children in any significant way. She died from sepsis, related to a urinary track infection, in the spring of 2009. She was 57 years old.

CHAPTER 3

THE SINGLE DAD

Steven's journey as a single parent began the day he was awarded custody of his two sons back in 1991. The boys were ages two and four, and quite a handful. Because my brother was a self-employed accountant he worked mostly from his home. This certainly made life a little easier for him, but his business was slow-growing, and at times he struggled to pay his bills. Within a year he decided to put his house up for sale and downsized to an apartment with a rental fee that was more affordable than his mortgage. I remember helping him pack up his house, and one memory will never leave me; the contents of a crawlspace under his home. It was a dark and dank space where my brother had never stored anything. But when I looked to make sure there was nothing in there I was stunned by a sea of empty rum bottles. He was quite shocked as well. And so we discovered where his wife tossed all her empty liquor bottles.

My brother and his boys settled comfortably in their new apartment. His younger son was always good- natured, responsible, honest, organized, and quite mature for his years. He was also a very kind and loving child, and an excellent student. Richard, although two years his senior, was quite the opposite. He was less mature, often angry, very forgetful, disorganized, and unfocused. He was also a poor student, and sadly, a chronic liar. Where his younger brother was always aware of what needed to be done, Richard lacked a sense of awareness and urgency regarding most situations. It was his younger brother who helped Richard get dressed, tie his shoes, and prepared his morning cereal. When there were chores to be done, Richard followed the instructions and example of his younger brother.

Richard's chronic lying became a very major concern for my brother. While his younger son was always open and honest about everything he thought and did, Richard could never be trusted. In fact, Richard was so incredibly convincing in his tales that I would classify him as an expert liar. If you asked Richard if he had any homework he would usually answer, "No," or "Yes, but I already did it." But if you demanded to see it you would discover nothing had been done. If you asked Richard how he did on an exam he would say, "really good," despite receiving a failing grade. My brother would call me frequently to complain about Richard's behavior and I would sympathize, always thinking how difficult it must be raising these two young boys by himself. So often he would say, "I worry about what will become of Richard."

During the times Steven had business conferences to attend, or just needed a little time for himself, I would take the boys. These were wonderful times for me because I enjoyed giving my nephews a little motherly love and attention. Of course, I didn't fret too much about their homework or messiness. I was their aunt and I just wanted to have fun with them and form good memories. I was always glad when I could give my brother a hand, and he was always so grateful.

In retrospect, I feel guilty when I remember some of the conversations I had with Steven regarding Richard. When he would call me to ventilate I would often respond by saying he needed to spend more time with Richard. His younger son was better adjusted and had many friends. Richard, however, was not well liked by his peers and always seemed to put himself directly in the path of calamity. I especially remember a shoplifting scheme that Richard set up in which he convinced his younger brother to participate. It was poorly executed and they got caught. Where his younger brother cried, apologized, and was devastated, it didn't faze Richard. Nothing ever seemed to bother Richard, and he never showed remorse.

Those were tough years for Steven, and I was proud of him. He was managing as best he could, and the boys were growing up despite all the challenges that presented. For example, Richard had a problem with sleepwalking and would wander outside the apartment in the middle of the night. Steven's solution was for the three of them to share one bed and put Richard in the middle. That way they could stop him when he tried to roam at night. And when Steven could not be home when the boys came home from school, he would make sure there were easy snacks in the cupboard and a routine to follow. But the stress was constant, and Steven's weight was a measure of his mood. He soothed his depression by extreme overeating and his obesity was becoming more and more dangerous to his health. When he met his second wife he was already weighing in at 250 pounds, and this weight was packed on his short 5'7" frame. Now, in 2001, he was surely a hundred pounds beyond that. During one of the weeks I was caring for the boys I remember my younger nephew saying to me, "Aunt Sherry, our Dad is so big and I am afraid he might die. If he dies what will become of us?" I responded by saying, "Don't worry, he'll be fine. But if something should ever happen, you will always have a home with us."

CHAPTER 4

SELF-DESTRUCTION

February 15, 2001 was a cold and dreary day. I was at work, knee-deep in the usual problems that I have to wrap my head around as a director in a large healthcare system. As I was preparing for my second meeting of the day, I received a call from a man who claimed to be a friend of my brother, and also one of his accounting clients. He stated that he had been meeting with Steven in regards to filing his income tax, and he believed that my brother had suffered a heart attack in his presence. He said he located my name and phone number from an emergency information contact card that was tucked away in my brother's wallet, and he told me Steven was alive when the ambulance arrived.

I was stunned. Despite knowing that my brother was at high risk for a cardiac event it still took me by surprise. After a moment of processing I became filled with a terrible feeling of dread. I then gathered myself together and hurried to where I was to meet with my staff that morning. I told them about the information I had just received and that I was heading to the hospital across town where Steven had been taken. I'll never forget my parting words, "I'll call you with an update after I arrive at the hospital, but somehow I feel my life will never be the same." And it never was.

When I arrived at the hospital, a facility that was part of the health system that employed me, I was greeted by a competent team of medical staff who knew me. They were expecting me and prepared, and I was emotionally distraught to say the least. I asked through my tears, "how is my brother doing? When can I see him?" The team, comprised of a social worker and nurse, silently and gently led me to a private room where the social worker explained that, despite all efforts to save my brother's life, he had died. So much emotion welled up inside of me. I wanted to see him, my only sibling; I wanted to be with him.

The nurse understood and gave me a tender hug. Then she took me to the room where my brother was being kept. There, on a stretcher, lying on his back, so quiet, so final. As uncontrollable tears flowed down my cheeks I thought to myself, "Why didn't you take better care of yourself? Your family needed you." With tubes remaining in his mouth, and his rotund body still warm, I climbed up beside him on the stretcher and hugged him tight. After a while I whispered these words to him, "Rest in peace, Steven. I loved you so much. You've worked hard in your life, and I know how much you struggled. I will take care of your boys now. Your job is done. I will miss you forever."

My brother was 53 years old, six years my senior. The scene was so surreal as I continued to lie with him on the stretcher. I felt frozen in time until finally the nurse came back to get me. She told me that the social worker was waiting for me back at the room where they had brought me initially. Slowly I sat up, kissed my brother a final goodbye on his cheek, and followed the nurse back. The social worker informed me that several of my brother's friends had arrived and wanted to help. Suddenly reality was setting in and I knew there was much to be done in very little time. My nephews were still in school, and dismissal time was only an hour away. The school must be called, and somehow arrangements would have to be made for someone to keep them until I could pick them up. I had to call my boss and staff to let them know what happened and when I might return to work. My parents lived in

Florida and must be notified. I had to call the funeral home. My head was spinning, my gut was churning, and I was barely thinking straight.

With the help of the hospital staff, and Steven's friends, everything came together. The calls were made and friends of my brother picked up my nephews from school, keeping them until I could get them later that evening. The call to my parents was especially hard, and I will never forget hearing my mother's sadness and sobs. They flew in the next morning ready to help with the funeral plans and with packing up Steven's apartment. My entire family came together to help, except for my husband, who was overseas at the time. My three adults children were especially quick to help in any way, and they were a Godsend for all the support they gave to their cousins.

It was a long and emotional time for all of us. According to Jewish custom, Steven was buried two days following his death, and a mourning period (Shiva) continued at my home for seven days. I took a three month leave of absence from my job so that we could all begin adjusting to our new normal. I also had to begin the legal guardianship process.

CHAPTER 5

GUARDIANSHIP

Oh how my life had changed! Adjusting to two active children, ages 11 and 13, who were grieving the loss of their father in a new living environment, was extremely challenging. And the bureaucratic system for seeking guardianship was hair-raising to say the least. The entire process, which involved detailed scrutiny by the Department of Social Services, and lengthy court system procedures, took about six months. Not to mention, that when all was said and done, my husband began complaining that he no longer wanted a part in raising my nephews. Initially, he was agreeable to share in the responsibility and guardianship, welcoming them into our home. But after he began experiencing their rambunctious behaviors he changed his tune and asked to have his name removed from the final guardianship papers. I will admit that Richard was especially challenging, but my disappointment in my husband created additional tension in our marriage, which was already on shaky ground.

My nephews did have an aunt (a sister to their mother) who also showed interest in becoming their guardian. In all fairness she could have provided a good home to them, but she did not live in their current school district and she did not know them very well. Social Services evaluated both of us for guardianship but ultimately thought my home was a better fit. This made me happy; my husband not so much.

All through the process of obtaining guardianship the boys lived with us. This was not legal but no one seemed to care. Their middle school worked with me and agreed that we should keep life as normal as possible for them. I was able to provide a large bedroom for them to share, and brought over some of their old furniture. They helped select fabric for new curtains, and in a few weeks they started to feel like they had a home again.

After their first month in our home, I arranged for the boys to see psychologists. They each had their own. Although I provided a lot of emotional support to them, I thought they would benefit from professional counseling to help them through their grieving process. And really, they had so much more to cope with than many children could even imagine. It was difficult not to feel sad for them with a cognitively impaired mother who was a ward of the state, and who they really never knew; and now with the loss of their father, the only security they had.

But we established a routine and the days went by. I became involved in their school activities, celebrated their birthdays, attended their sports events, had their friends over, carpooled them to social events, and just gave them lots of love. In six months I was back to work, but I was never the same. I had never worked full time when my own children were that young and it was a struggle. Raising a second family is a lot of work, especially without the emotional and physical support of your spouse.

CHAPTER 6

UNRAVELING THE MYSTERY

Life went along fairly bump-free for my younger nephew. He always took everything in stride; a very resilient child. After several therapy sessions he bounced back, re-adjusted to school, and re-connected with his friends. He was extremely well liked by both his peer group and his teachers. He excelled in school and enjoyed his popularity. He was a natural athlete, incredibly charismatic, and very mature for his age of eleven years.

If my younger nephew had any shortcomings I would have to say it was his forgetfulness. For the most part this was comical. But at times it was very frustrating; lost watches, jackets, hats, gloves, books, and even backpacks can become annoying over time. But he had such a winning way with people and an incredible upbeat perspective on life. Despite his orphaned status he considered himself "the luckiest kid in the world." And when it came to helping with Richard he was invaluable.

Richard was a different story. It didn't take more than a few days after having him move in to see that something was not quite right with Richard. All those memories of conversations I had with my brother were coming back to haunt me. I used to think that if my brother would just give Richard more attention, and spend more quality time with him, that it would go a long way in solving most of the problems he had with Richard. But I soon discovered, that despite giving Richard so much of my time, his behaviors remained the same.

Richard was a puzzle to us all. I believed for a while that his problems were mostly emotional. After all, not having a nurturing mother in his life, losing his father, and adjusting to a whole new environment could adversely affect anyone. Therefore, although I stopped my younger nephew's therapy sessions, I continued to take Richard weekly to the child psychologist. This was a struggle as Richard put up a fight every week, but somehow I convinced him to get in the car.

Over time, the psychologist thought he had established a good relationship with Richard, and after several months diagnosed him with Oppositional Behavioral Disorder (OBD). As a mental health professional myself, I did not agree, although some elements of this diagnosis were a good fit with Richard's behavior. For example, he would not listen to reason or authority figures (myself, teachers, other family members, etc.) and could get rather angry if made to do something he did not want to do. This applied to doing his homework, brushing his teeth, going to bed at night, and anything else he might disagree with. Richard was also a pathological liar, and a good one at that. He always spun such a good tale, that if you didn't know his history, you would easily believe him. He hated going to school and rarely did homework or completed assignments. Of course if asked whether he did his homework he would always say yes and show you something that might pass for homework. But one call to the teacher would always confirm his dishonesty. Richard could never, ever be trusted to tell the truth.

There were so many other behaviors that just didn't fit the OBD diagnosis. For one thing, Richard had very little awareness of events going on around him, or even of his own surroundings. He would walk across the street and not even think about the possibility of a car coming. He never even looked to see if a car was coming. Several times he almost got hit and he thought it was funny. Richard could be a block away from home and have no idea where he was. He had absolutely no concept of time, and he never mastered the skill of telling time. Show him an analog watch and he was bewildered. He could read numbers on a digital watch, but he relied on his brother to wake him in the morning, advise him when it was bedtime, and even when to leave the house to catch the school bus in the morning. When Richard moved up to the high school and had a later bus then his brother in middle school, he would miss the bus unless I reminded him to get out on the bus stop. Often I thought he had left for the bus only to find him still in his room. Too many times I had to drive him to school. Too many times he caused me to be late for work. Too many times I thought the stress would incapacitate me.

And there were other unusual and behaviors. Mealtimes were especially challenging because Richard had no concept of portion control. Left unchecked, he would eat every food item placed on the table despite knowing that food would need to be shared with others. I learned quickly that I could not set out a platter of fried chicken without Richard grabbing the lion's share. When it came to food he had little regard for the rest of the family, and his appetite was truly insatiable. His understanding of a normal serving size was just not there, so it was necessary to be specific as to what he could have. You would think that Richard could learn in time that two chicken breasts was his portion, or two hamburgers, etc. But this was never the case. As with everything else, Richard had a poor memory. He also lacked judgement and insight. Despite repetitive training, the outcome was always the same. He could not remember from day to day, and he was incapable of learning from cause and effect.

Regardless of Richards's shortcomings, he was smart in many ways. He could understand and play computer games for hours on end, and he could understand and enjoy many movies. In fact, he was tested by several psychologists and determined to be in the average range of intelligence. One psychologist had stated that, "Richard functions in an average range of intellectual ability, but his working memory is quite limited, and his orientation is problematic." The psychologist concluded that Richard had a learning disability and a language processing deficit. So despite Richard testing in the normal intelligence range, he could never remember his date of birth, the date of Christmas, who was President of the United States, or even what season it was.

When it came to the concept of money, Richard was totally lost. Early on I learned never to give him more than a few dollars. Once I gave him a ten dollar bill to purchase a doughnut. When I asked him for the change he replied, "What change?" He had given the bill over and walked away immediately after receiving the food. I was amazed that a fifteen year old boy could have so little knowledge about the value of a dollar and what it could buy; nor could he understand the concept of saving money.

Then there was the problem concerning Richard's eyes. The school reported that he did not pass the vision test. I actually had noticed that he would often squint and hold papers and objects directly in front of his nose in order to view them. But when questioned about his ability to see he would vehemently deny having any sight issues. Now with the school report to confirm my suspicions, I scheduled an optometrist appointment. When Richard started to complain, his brother told me that he had worn glasses in the past but that he would always lose them, and that finally his father stopped replacing them.

Sure enough, the optometry exam revealed that Richard was extremely near-sighted and should be wearing glasses all the time. So began the challenge of keeping Richard in glasses, and I soon realized why my brother just gave up the fight.

Almost as challenging was the battle to convince Richard to dress appropriately during the cold winter months. This struggle was so difficult because Richard never took note of the weather or seasons. He actually dressed as if every day was a summer day. Cold temperatures never phased him. He loved his tee-shirts and shorts, and if I did not pay close attention to his daily attire he would run out of the house in a snowstorm dressed for a hot summer day. The winter coat fight became so frustrating and tiresome as he absolutely hated to wear one. When I insisted he wear a coat to school it usually did not come home with him. Endless trips were made to the school's Lost and Found, and it was rare that coats and eyeglasses were ever seen again.

In addition to Richard's high tolerance to cold, he had an unusually high pain threshold. Sometimes he would accidentally bump his head hard while getting into the car and he wouldn't experience any discomfort; or he would scrape his knee on concrete from a fall and never complain of pain. It was incredible how much pain Richard could withstand, so when he asked if he could get a tattoo for his sixteenth birthday I decided to allow him to get a modest one on his shoulder blade. He selected a simple scorpion image and I took him to a reputable tattoo studio that I was familiar with. I explained to him what he might feel in regards to the tattooing process and he said he was not afraid, and that he was ready and excited. When the tattoo artist began working on the tattoo Richard did not even flinch. In fact, he said that he hardly felt a thing. Just like frigid weather had no effect on him, neither did the tattoo needles.

Going out with Richard to eat at a restaurant was another curious yet predictable experience. He could read words but his ability to comprehend was lacking. So when a menu was placed in his hands he could never figure out how to make sense of it, or understand what food items were available. He would pick up the menu and his eyes would dart everywhere. It was too much for him to process, however, if there was a picture he would be drawn to select it as his choice. He could never understand the format of a menu (appetizers, entrees, sides, deserts, etc.). Most of the time he would wait for his brother, or one of his cousins to order, and then he would say, "I'll take that, too."

Another problem that Richard exhibited was his inability to stay awake while being a passenger in a car. This may not seem like a serious situation, but it complicated my ability to help him learn about his local surroundings. Within a few minutes of my driving he would always nod out, and this interfered with teaching him geographical awareness. I would be explaining to Richard about different landmarks to help him with street recognition in our neighborhood, and then I would realize he had fallen asleep.

The behaviors mentioned thus far are only the tip of the iceberg. There was the horrific incident when Richard befriended a pedophile he had met in a chat room on the internet. I overheard him talking in his room to someone on the phone. The conversation appeared to be about homosexual foreplay. When questioned about who he was speaking with he responded, "just a friend." But then later that day the man called our home and my husband answered. The caller thought it was Richard and began talking to him in a seductive manner, requesting sexual acts.

When I confronted Richard about the call he admitted that he had become friendly with this man in a chat room and that the man had a similar background as him. Apparently they had been discussing their life situation and the man told Richard that his mother was also impaired and living in a nursing home. He also told Richard that his father had died of a heart attack. Now I could see how easily Richard had been comforted by this stranger, and it was difficult for me to get upset with him knowing how naive he was.

Yes, Richard was the epitome of naivety. Even more worrisome, he exhibited a total lack of anxiety towards strangers. If I was out shopping with Richard I could not take my eyes off him. This was not an easy task as he had a strong tendency to wander away, and a total lack of fearfulness. He would act impulsively, disappearing quickly if I got distracted. Taking him out in any public situation was challenging as he required my undivided attention. Left unwatched he was also prone to shoplifting. He would remove items from shelves and slip them in his pockets. When caught and asked why he took something he would respond, "Because I wanted it." There was never any remorse. A super ego was truly absent in Richard.

The most frustrating problem with Richard was that he could never learn from his mistakes. As a result, he would continue to make the same mistakes over and over and over again. Richard was just incapable of seeing the relationship between cause and effect. A simple deduction, like how taking a very long shower would deplete the hot water supply for the rest of the family, was impossible for him to make. Or that over-loading the washing machine would result in malfunction. And not picking up rocks on the lawn before mowing would damage the mower deck. The list is endless. The family turmoil and frustration that resulted from Richard's lack of insight and judgment was ongoing, and always at a high level.

But of all the problems I faced with Richard, the most disheartening was his poor school performance. While all three of my own children graduated from the same high school that Richard was attending, I never knew there was a school psychologist or a special team of educators for children with special needs. This was all so new to me, and in my opinion, the team just didn't understand Richard's problems. Yes, they tried to follow a process and developed what they called an "Individualized Education Plan (IEP)," but the plan was so flawed in meeting his needs, and the outcome was so poor for Richard. Despite my spending many hours at the school meeting with his team, no improvement could be noted in his school work. Richard was supposed to bring home daily reports for me to sign, but he could never remember to bring them home, or find them. He was placed in a special class with two teachers, however, he never realized there were two teachers in the room; nor could he remember any teacher's names. Despite the efforts made to improve his academic performance, summer school was always necessary, and he did poorly in those classes as well, although he was given passing grades to move him along.

I felt like I was at my rope's end. Totally exhausted, frustrated, and struggling to keep my marriage afloat, I called a close friend, a teacher, just to ventilate and toss ideas around. Why wasn't the school able to help Richard more? Could he really be a hopeless case? I just thought I was missing something. My friend and I spoke at length about the behavioral and academic problems Richard exhibited, and then she suggested a book for me to read called, ***The Broken Cord***, by Michael Dorris. She explained it was a true story about a Native American child with similar problems as Richard, and that it might be helpful. I was open to anything- any tips, any insight, that might help me understand more about Richard.

I purchased the book and started reading. My first thought was about how the young child in the story was much more impaired intellectually, and more regressed, than Richard. I didn't see a connection at first, but I read on. The story was heart-wrenching, about a single father who adopted a Native American child (Adam) with a multitude of developmental, intellectual, and behavioral deficits. The more I read, the more I began to notice incredible similarities in how Adam and Richard reacted to life situations, problem-solved, and in their physical appearance as well. Although Adam had a lower IQ than Richard, their behaviors in so many areas were the same. Halfway through the book I realized, beyond a doubt, that Richard had some degree of Fetal Alcohol Syndrome (FAS). Reading this book resulted in the ultimate "A-ha" moment for me. This feeling, of finally knowing what was wrong with Richard, was exhilarating! Although the book was actually quite pessimistic about successful behavioral management for this diagnosis, I didn't let that discourage me. Knowledge is power, and I felt on top of the world.

CHAPTER 7

FAMILY IMPACT

Now that I had some answers I was fresh with enthusiasm on my crusade to get help for Richard. I was reassured in some ways by the fact that Richard's behaviors were by no fault of his own. I was determined, more than ever, to make a meaningful difference in his life, and to help pave a way forward for him so that he could be assured of a positive and successful future. Unfortunately, all of my family did not share or embrace my eagerness and optimism.

My husband was the most intolerant of Richard. He wasn't especially fond of my younger nephew either, but Richard was always the most challenging and therefore the greatest bone of contention. My husband despised all the time and effort I devoted to Richard in regards to working with his school problems, and he was resentful of Richard's inability to take on responsibilities around the home. Richard had a way of breaking everything he touched which further fanned the fire. My husband was always pleading for me to give my nephews over to social services, but I never considered this as an option. The situation put such a wedge in our relationship that marriage counseling became a necessity.

My three children, now all young adults and still living at home, were much better in accepting and adjusting to our new living situation. I tried hard to instill in them the importance of caring for family, and certainly some of this took hold. After all, I loved my nephews, and our home was the most stable and logical place for them to live. I also loved my brother, and I could feel his presence and appreciation knowing that his boys were well cared for. I am proud of my children as they all made sacrifices and rose to the occasion. My oldest son gave up his bedroom for my nephews to share, and he moved into my daughter's room. My daughter moved into our guest room. The entire family was affected, and everyone made concessions and took on new responsibilities. My husband, however, continued to struggle, acting violently to the suggestion of giving up the guest room for our daughter to use. I still remember his shouting, his cruel words echo in my mind to this very day, "I don't want your nephews here. I shouldn't have to bear the burden of your brother's irresponsible and reckless lifestyle!"

Through all the turmoil, I continued to have Richard evaluated by professionals to determine his eligibility for more appropriate services. Public school had very little to offer, and what they did offer just wasn't working. The evaluation process was lengthy and expensive. Richard was evaluated by an independent psychologist, the Maryland State Department of Education Division of Rehabilitation Services (DORS), the Maryland Department of Health and Mental Hygiene, and the Kennedy Krieger Institute Department of Neuropsychology at Johns Hopkins. But because Richard was able to present himself well, and tested low normal on a battery of IQ tests, he was deemed ineligible for immediate developmental disability services. The encouraging news was that Richard was determined to have the highest level of disability by DORS (Category I: Individuals with the Most Significant Disabilities) and would be eligible for vocational rehabilitation services after completion of high school. This would ensure job training and living assistance post graduation.

Meanwhile, the strain continued in my marriage, and this did not go unnoticed by my nephews. Richard had mentioned a desire to attend a military school several months back, and suddenly this did not sound like such a bad idea to me. True, it wouldn't address his learning and behavioral issues, but maybe the structure would be good for him. Upon graduation he could proceed with the DORS vocational rehabilitation plan. My husband was certainly in favor of this plan, and I thought it might help save my marriage. I was wrong on this calculation. In the end, my husband sought out an old high school crush and then left me for her. He said, "You chose your nephews; this is the price."

So, for my own sanity, I began to research military schools.

CHAPTER 8

A MANAGEABLE PATH

Not knowing where to start, I went where I usually begin— on the internet. None of my friends or family members could make any recommendations so this seemed as good as any place to check on what military schools were out there… and it was. There were numerous schools to look at, and the task was actually overwhelming. I limited my search by location and cost and there were still so many. My husband was unwilling to spend any of his income on Richard's schooling so I was bound by the Social Security Income (SSI) that I received for his care. I was hoping to find a school close by to us in Maryland, but affordability was an issue. Finally, I discovered a school in Pennsylvania which was about a three hour drive from our home. This school seemed to meet most of my criteria; it was small, accredited, had good reviews, and within my budget.

I printed out the school's information from their website and shared it with Richard. He was extremely excited about the idea of attending a military school, but he was incapable of really comprehending what it would fully mean in regards to a life change. Richard gazed at the pictures, stared in awe at the uniforms and marching videos, but the information about academic expectations and the rigid daily schedule were just words on a page to him. But he was so ecstatic at the mere thought of attending a military school! So we completed an application, and I scheduled an appointment for us to meet with the Head Master and begin the interview process.

It was the 2001-2002 winter break for the public schools in Baltimore. Richard had already made his way through one quarter of ninth grade with barely-passing grades. If everything worked out as I had hoped, Richard would complete ninth grade at the military school and continue through graduation.

The military school visit was a family event. All of us went, including my husband (he didn't leave me until November 2002). The campus was old, quaint, and inviting, and reminded me of a small college. Richard was somewhat curious, but the rest of us were very interested and excited, taking note of the school environment. Still, my largest concern was that Richard might not get accepted into the school. His grade average was extremely low, D+ at best. And there was an admission exam in addition to the personal interview. There would also be reference checks from a few of Richard's teachers which I could only pray would be positive.

Looking back, we must have looked like such a motley crew; a troop of seven, with Richard and I leading the way. We were greeted by a student who was dressed in the military school uniform, a very polite young man. He seated all of us in the Head Master's office where we waited only a few minutes before a tall and powerful-looking man entered and greeted us. Indeed, the Head master appeared to be someone you would not want to disagree with! He introduced himself with a strong Spanish accent, "I am Colonel Diego," and shook all of our hands.

The Colonel put us all at ease quite quickly. Despite his stern appearance, he exhibited a gentleness that made him very likable. We all sat and listened as the Colonel spoke about the school. For about twenty minutes he spoke about the school's history, then he moved into specifics about the curriculum for at least another twenty minutes, and then he rounded out the hour by talking about what he called, "a day in the life of a military student," which pretty much described a typical day from sunrise to bedtime.

The Colonel proceeded to pull out a folder that contained information I had mailed previously. Among the documents were responses from the teacher references that I had provided, Richard's grade reports from the past few years, his most recent annual medical report, and a paper that I completed as Richard's legal guardian that provided a little personal background information. When the Colonel remarked about Richard's poor grades I felt my anxiety rise. Then Richard blurted out, "Yeah, I know I'm not the best student, and I'm not super smart, but I don't study like I should." If the Colonel was disappointed, it did not show on his face. Then he talked with Richard about how difficult it must be losing a father. Richard just nodded his head. Then the Colonel sent all of my family out to walk around the campus for an hour so he could talk with Richard in private, and also to administer the pre-admission exam.

When our family returned to the Colonel's office Richard had just completed the exam. He looked exhausted, and all of us were pretty tired as well. It was a long day for sure. I asked Richard what he thought of the exam and he said, "it was okay; just a lot of questions," The Colonel left us all waiting in his office for about another twenty minutes or so, and when he returned he asked to speak with me alone. So I followed the Colonel into another private office. He closed the door and we both sat facing each other, my anxiety escalating.

The Colonel remarked, "Richard has had a tough life." He then went on to say, "his math and grammar skills are poor, and I can't say with any certainty that he will do well here academically. We have students here with learning disabilities and we work hard with them to build skills. But on questions that measure confidence and self-esteem Richard scored especially poor, and in these areas I truly believe our school can make a difference. At least I'd like to give it a try."

I was so happy at hearing these words that I cried tears of joy. I felt so grateful that Richard had been accepted into the school, and maybe, just maybe, he would succeed here. I stood up and said, "Thank you, Sir," and shook his hand. Then the Colonel handed me an envelope with more forms to complete, and a list of items that Richard would need to bring with him when he reported to the school in just two weeks. Then he said, "Lets tell Richard!"

CHAPTER 9

DRIVER'S ED

Richard was fifteen years old and about midway through ninth grade when he entered the military school. It was a blessing for me. I felt like a great load had been lifted from my back. No more struggles getting Richard out the door in the morning to catch the school bus, no more daily visits to the high school, and no more arguments about completing homework. I also could stop my worrying about the severity of punishments I would dole out (all ineffective) for his negative behaviors such as lying, stealing, smoking marijuana, insubordination, etc. Although Richard would still be home for holidays and summer breaks, this would at least be manageable.

There were still problems with Richard, but the military school was quite tolerant. For example, Richard continued to lose belongings at an alarming rate. But as long as I kept sending money to cover the replacement costs for items such as pieces of his uniform (often belt buckles and shoes), school supplies, personal toiletries, etc., they could accept this persistent behavior. At some point both the school and I agreed it was impossible to keep up with his need for eyeglass replacement so we let this go. And academically, Richard continued to require summer school, which kept him at the school during most of the summer break.

I did make routine trips to the school to meet with Richard's teachers and also to watch him march in the annual parades. I was so pleased at how well he adjusted to the structured school routine, and how proud he was when he was marching in uniform. The Colonel was right when he said the school might improve Richard's self-esteem. I could see it in his face and posturing, and for the first time Richard had friends!

When Richard came home during his first winter break we were all so excited to see him. My husband was no longer around to complain (November 2002 marked our legal separation), and his brother and cousins were looking forward to the family reunion. My daughter made the journey with me to pick him up from the school (as she often did), and Richard fell asleep in the car during the ride home (as always).

As we pulled up in front of our home, Richard was eager to play all his favorite computer games. He ignored all requests to help carry in his belongings and ran straight into the house. My daughter and I were left with the task of bringing in all his gear (no surprise). Despite Richard saying he would sort out his dirty laundry and school assignments later, this never happened. My daughter and I ended up washing and re-packing his clothing, and the schoolwork assignments to be completed over the break never got a look. This became the regular routine during all of Richard's school breaks.

Richard was approaching sixteen, and like most teenagers, he wanted to drive. Needless to say, I was horrified at the thought. Despite Richard's shortcomings, he thought of himself as a normal and capable person. I was reluctant to allow him to get a learner's permit which made him extremely angry. He yelled and carried on, accusing me of treating him like "a retard." Deep within my heart I trusted my decision, but Richard continued to persist in his pursuit of wanting to drive. He would not let up, and as a result I began to feel guilty, actually doubting my decision. To help better guide me, I called Richard's medical doctor for advice. After a lengthy conversation about Richard's capabilities his physician said this, "Richard is not stupid, and kids with lower IQs have been able to master the skill of driving. I think you should consider giving him a chance." And so I did.

I downloaded the study guide posted by the Motor Vehicle Administration (MVA) and gave it to Richard so that he could begin studying the rules of the road. He was beyond excited! Richard had a smile that could warm your heart, and his enthusiasm brought me a feeling of new hope. Maybe Richard was more capable than I gave him credit for? I had experienced this feeling before, only to end up so disappointed. Maybe this time would be different.

After a few days Richard said he was ready to take the written driving test. A passing score on this test would allow him to receive the learner's permit. I drove him to the MVA, all the while feeling cautiously optimistic. To my pleasant surprise, Richard passed the test! He got three answers wrong, the lowest passing score, but he passed. Richard was beaming with pride, and I was really proud of him. I still harbored feelings of ambivalence, but this was great for his self-esteem.

When we returned home, all of the family was so thrilled for him. I called my car insurance company and had Richard added to the policy. Then I took him out for his first road lesson. Richard was raring to go, thinking he could just take off. But I kept the experience limited to just a few neighborhood roads, and he actually did okay. I remember thinking that maybe this will work out just fine. If nothing else, seeing that smile on Richard's face was amazing!

Unfortunately, day two of Richard on the road was not so positive. For one thing, he was extremely cocky. He didn't want to listen to anything I had to say. He would drive too fast, keep only one hand on the steering wheel, and most distressing, he was not recognizing the road signs. When he drove through the first stop sign I began to worry. When he didn't understand what a "yield" sign meant my concern grew. But when Richard insisted on going in reverse at a stop sign, without looking in the rear view mirror, I knew all was not going well. In an instant he crashed into a car behind us, putting my anxiety level off the chart. The driver behind us came out yelling, unable to understand why his car was slammed into. Despite all my apologies, and explaining to him that Richard was a new student driver, the man remained irate. Richard just sat in the car, not really understanding what went wrong. After the transfer of insurance information I drove us home.

That was my last time driving with Richard. I decided my nerves just couldn't take it. So I enlisted the help of my three adult children to take him out on the road. One by one they each drove with him and came back with their own horror stories. In the end, we all decided that it was not safe to allow Richard to drive. Needless to say, Richard was furious. But this time I held firm to my beliefs, and I know it was the right decision.

My relationship was never the same with Richard after the failed driving experience. No matter how I tried to explain my feelings, he felt that he had been severely wronged. I would tell him how much I loved him and feared for his safety, and he would turn it around by saying, "you just hate me, that's all." Sometimes I felt so crushed by his remarks, but I stood my ground on the driving. I tried to make it up to Richard in other ways, such as buying him a new computer, writing him more frequently, responding more quickly to any requests he made, but it was clear that our relationship was deteriorating.

CHAPTER 10

COMING OF AGE

During Richard's last two years at the military school he had become very close friends with a fellow student. This student had been his roommate, and they shared a brother-like bond. In fact, Richard had spent his last two winter breaks with his friend's family up in Connecticut. This family had become rather fond of Richard, claiming he was like a second son to them. I admit to being skeptical about them, knowing how difficult Richard could be. But I was also grateful that Richard had such a good friend, something he never had when he was living with me and attending public school.

Meanwhile, I was becoming increasingly worried about what path Richard's future would take. He was quickly approaching eighteen, and I would be facing a court hearing soon about the possible termination of his guardianship. I was also beginning to make plans with the Maryland DORS program in hopes of securing a residential and vocational employment opportunity for Richard. They had previously deemed him eligible for services upon high school graduation. The good news was that DORS had placed Richard on a waiting list for independent housing in an apartment building, and had lined up an excellent job opportunity for him, working on computers, with job coaching. It looked like a good plan and that things were starting to shape up.

But my optimism was short-lived. Richard was not on board with this plan. He did not like the idea of taking a bus to work and "having someone looking over him on the job." Instead, he wanted to move in with his friend in Connecticut right after graduation, and find a job close to their home. He was dead-set on this arrangement and told me I couldn't stop him. So I called Richard's friend's mother to verify that they wanted Richard to live with them and to further assess the feasibility of this arrangement.

The family appeared to be caring and genuine in their affection towards Richard. They confirmed that they wanted Richard to stay with them stating, "Richard is like another son to us, and we will look after him." The mother said she was preparing a room for Richard and that it would also be beneficial to their son to have him living there. I expressed my desire to keep Richard in Maryland and explained what services he had qualified for. But the friend's mother did not appear to see Richard's shortcomings, and believed his needs would be adequately met living with her family in Connecticut.

Maybe I was mistaken, but I sensed a coolness about this woman. I know that Richard did not speak kindly of me to her, and I felt that she believed I was not looking out for his best interest. I was very open with her about Richard's FAS, but she did not seem concerned in the least. She said she would help Richard seek employment, start a savings account, and encourage him to further his education when he was ready. I explained that it would be difficult to keep Richard on track with any plan, and that he would need a lot of supervision, but she was not deterred. In the end I went along with this plan as there really was no way for me to stop it. But I made one request of this woman, "Please don't let Richard drive." I explained my family's experience with Richard behind the wheel and how we all believed, deep in our hearts, that it would be dangerous to let him drive. I told her that if he was to drive I believed it would result in his death, and possibly someone else's as well.

In the meantime, Richard's senior year seemed to be speeding along. I was becoming anxious about his upcoming guardianship hearing that was scheduled the week he would turn eighteen. At the same time, I was feeling so very weary. It seemed that every day I would receive word from the school about lost items I needed to pay for. It was so constant that I began waiting until the end of each week before sending money. Sometimes I was asked to just replace the lost items (i.e.; toothbrushes, hair combs, soap) in lieu of money. Whether sending money or replacing lost things, it became so tiresome.

Finally the guardianship court hearing was before us. I picked up Richard from the school and we drove, mostly in silence, to the late afternoon hearing. The court-appointed lawyer was required to investigate whether there was "clear and convincing evidence that cause exists to continue the appointment of a guardian." He began by reviewing all of Richard's psychological evaluation reports. Then he met with Richard and I, both together and separately. Finally, the lawyer spoke with the family in Connecticut over telephone.

The lawyer's investigative report and conclusions were mind-boggling to me. The psychological evaluation that documented Richard's limited working memory, problematic orientation, and language processing deficit had little bearing because his IQ was noted to be in the average range. Richard's comments about wanting to be independent, and stating that I under-estimated his abilities, seemed to far outweigh my reporting of his serious deficiencies. And the comments from Richard's friend's family, based on their limited time with Richard during two Christmas holidays, disputed my assessment of Richard's capabilities. The final court conclusion was, "There is not clear and convincing evidence that cause exists to continue the guardianship over Richard. Average intellectual ability does not require a life involving loss of control over your person and property. Society must be very careful before it imposes burdens on individual freedom."

Not a very thorough investigation to remove guardianship! Why didn't the lawyer question my three adult children, Richard's brother, or Richard's grandparents? These were the individuals who knew him best. I still am stunned that the friend's family was given such a high level of credibility while members of Richard's immediate family were completely left out of the investigation. Needless to say, I felt totally let down by the legal system, and I feared for Richard's future. But Richard was thrilled, and began firming up his plans to move in with his friend right after graduation. He was not even coming home.

Graduation day came just a few weeks later, and our entire family attended this special day. We were beaming with pride over Richard, so proud that he was able to make it this far. It was a long day, but one we will always remember and cherish. All of us went out to dinner after the ceremonies were finished, and we returned Richard to the school where his friend, and friend's parents, were waiting. The family had packed up all of Richard's belongings in their car, and were eager to leave for their home in Connecticut. We gave Richard our final good luck wishes and hugs, encouraged him to use his savings wisely (money that I had put away for him), and told him we would be in touch frequently. That was the last time we saw Richard alive.

CHAPTER 11

LIVES CUT SHORT

None of us heard much from Richard after graduation. He settled into his new home in Connecticut and appeared content in his new surroundings. Richard and his friend remained very close, and for that I was grateful. Richard called to let me know he was job hunting, and this sparked a glimmer of hope in me, thinking that maybe he will start to make a place for himself in the world. My oldest son maintained the most contact with Richard. He had taken him under his wing early on, and they developed a close relationship. My son was planning his wedding for the following summer and they had asked Richard to be a groomsman. So there were several calls made between them to discuss the wedding plans.

Richard kept in touch with me primarily through e-mail. He rarely returned my phone calls, and I could feel that he continued to harbor resentment towards me. But he did manage to keep me up to date on his job status, which changed frequently. During Richard's eight months in Connecticut he went through four jobs. The first two jobs were with construction companies. Then he worked for American Eagle Outfitters. His last job was with Walmart. When I questioned him about each job loss he always had a story, and of course, it was never his fault. My optimism was beginning to dwindle.

By far the most frightening information I received from Richard was the news of his obtaining his driver's license. He used part of his savings to purchase a used car. His new family had not heeded my warning, and although I was devastated, I cannot say that I was surprised. The relationship between his friend's parents and myself was ice cold. I had always felt that they did not take my concerns about Richard seriously, and now this was confirmed. I can't say that I blame them a hundred percent as Richard could present himself as quite normal. His deficits were not readily visible, even by psychologists. Richard had clearly made a great impression with this family and had won them over. He could lie better than anyone I ever knew, and no doubt, his new family thought I was the evil aunt that Richard described so believably.

Upon hearing the news of Richard now driving, I began to re-evaluate and question my beliefs. Maybe he was truly capable of driving responsibly and safely? Maybe I had misjudged his comprehension and ability? But no matter how I tried to re-think the situation I still came up with the same conclusion. It was like a Pavlovian response, and I would not let myself be gaslighted. Every time I visualized Richard behind the steering wheel my stomach knotted up, and a sense of dread overtook me. No... this was not good news.

A couple of weeks after Richard began driving came news of his first accident. He had been driving home from work and hit a parked car. Apparently, Richard had fallen asleep at the wheel. His car was totaled, but no one was hurt. I had hoped this would curtail his driving, but his friend's parents decided to sell Richard one of their used vehicles. Then, a couple of months later, came news of Richard's second accident, a crash that again totaled his car. Luckily, no one was injured.

Still determined to get back on the road, Richard used the remainder of his savings to purchase a third car, a Ford Probe. This car was his pride and joy. He sent me several pictures of it, and in every one he was beaming from ear-to-ear. But my fears only continued to escalate. This was his third car in six months, and I was scared to death. There is nothing worse than knowing that a situation is dangerous, and there is nothing you can do about it.

The next few weeks were uneventful. I hadn't heard from Richard, but that was not unusual. Still, I couldn't help but worry about him. I had such an unsettling feeling, and Connecticut seemed so far away. My oldest son had spoken with him recently about his wedding plans, and Richard would be traveling to our town soon for his wedding. In just four months we would all get to see Richard again… or so we thought.

It was February 26, 2006. I had worked long and hard that day, and was in bed by 10 pm. When the phone rang at midnight I was in a deep sleep. I fumbled for the phone and forced out a weak 'Hello." The man on the other end, the father of Richard's friend, replied, "Sherry, I'm so sorry to have to tell you that Richard died tonight in a car accident." I jolted upright in bed, my worst fear realized. I asked for the details and cried.

It was a gruesome accident. A head-on collision that killed Richard and an unsuspecting young man, due to Richard's reckless driving. Richard was speeding down the highway, and proceeded to pass a tractor-trailer despite being in a no passing zone. He crossed over the double yellow line and collided with a driver coming in the opposite direction. Both were killed on contact, and pronounced dead at the crash scene. My poor nephew, a casualty of impulsive, irrational, and in-the-moment FAS behavior. And the other casualty, a responsible and loving husband and father, who just happened to be in the wrong place at the wrong time. Such a tragedy, one that I saw coming but was helpless to prevent.

I was numb. I was angry. It was difficult for me to think and process. My heart was aching. It was my greatest fear come reality. I wanted to scream obscenities at the family caring for Richard, but to what end? It was done. Richard's short life had come to an end, and another man was sacrificed. What good would the blame-game do at this point? I told the friend's father that I would make the funeral arrangements and have Richard's body returned to Baltimore. Richard would be buried next to his father.

And so my grieving process began. Five years after burying my brother I was placing his eldest son in the ground beside him. My brother's words resounded in my head, "What will become of Richard?" No need to ponder for an answer to that anymore.

Richard may be gone, but I will never forget him. Despite his shortcomings, he was a sensitive and loving child. His imperfections were through no fault of his own, and I have vowed to educate society about Fetal Alcohol Syndrome for the rest of my life.

CHAPTER 12

LESSONS LEARNED

In my crusade to educate the public about FAS, I have learned the following:

- Too many people do not believe that alcohol, even in small amounts, can result in fetal brain damage.

- FAS damage occurs on a continuum. In other words, the more a woman drinks during her pregnancy, the more brain damage (deficits) will be apparent in the child.

- A woman should cease to drink if she is trying to conceive. If she consumes alcohol up until the point that the pregnancy is confirmed her baby may already have some degree of FAS.

- *Fetal Alcohol Syndrome* (FAS), the most commonly used diagnosis, has many names. A less severe syndrome may be called *Fetal Alcohol Effect* (FAE). More comprehensive names include *Fetal Alcohol Spectrum Disorders* (FASD) and *Alcohol Related Neurological Disorders* (ARND).

- FAS warnings are usually placed in very obscure locations where alcohol is sold or served.

- Persons with FAS can have a normal IQ, and these individuals can be the most dangerous because their deficits are not easily recognizable. These persons can have a deadly impact on others.

- Children with FAS may, or may not, exhibit specific physical facial features such as narrow eyes, short nose, thin upper lip, pointed chin, and ear abnormalities, which are more evident between the ages of 8 months to 8 years.

- Severe behavioral problems are common in children with FAS. The symptoms are often diagnosed as Attention Deficit Disorder or Oppositional Disorder.

- If you see a pregnant woman drinking, educate her gently. Be prepared for her rejection of the facts.

- FAS is under-diagnosed, and often not recognized by medical or mental health professionals.

- Persons with FAS have difficulty recognizing the relationship between cause and effect. Therefore, they continue to make the same mistakes over and over again.

- Many prisoners in our penal system have some degree of FAS which makes their rehabilitation very challenging (due to inability to correlate cause and effect).

- *The Center for Disease Control* (CDC) provides free flyers, brochures, and posters that can be easily downloaded or ordered online. Despite this availability, many physicians do not display or provide information on the dangers of prenatal alcohol consumption.

- Many physicians, despite the evidence, still believe that it is safe to drink in moderation when pregnant. Remember: the severity of deficiencies is related to the amount of alcohol consumed.

- FAS is **not** reversible. It is permanent brain damage.

- There is a high percentage of FAS among children awaiting adoption. Parents-to-be should find out as much as possible about the birth mother before the adoption is final.

- Alcohol is a teratogen and therefore more permanently harmful to the developing baby. Babies exposed to marijuana, cocaine and heroin in the womb do not suffer permanent physical or cognitive effects.

- Raising a child with FAS will take a great toll on the family.

ADDENDUM

Eulogy

Photos of Richard (Baby and Adult)

Photo of Richard's Car After Fatal Crash

Surgeon General's Advisory on Alcohol Use in Pregnancy

Warnings on Alcoholic Beverages

Warning Sign Posted in Bar

CDC FAS Brochure

CDC FAS Poster

EULOGY FOR RICHARD

March 2, 2006

I want to take this moment to tell you a little bit about my nephew, Richard; to honor his very short life, to tell you all how special he was.

Richard, as some of you know, was a victim of Fetal Alcohol Syndrome, a condition that is 100 percent preventable, yet when it presents, it is 100 percent permanent and irreversible. Richard struggled with this disability, and I struggled with my feelings, thinking every day about how very sad and unfair his situation was through no fault of his own.

Richard's affliction was not readily visible, a blessing in many ways as it did not easily set him apart from others. But unfortunately, this allowed others to think him far more capable than he was. I will always marvel at how Richard set up my computer, yet remembering the date of his birthday presented a challenge for him. Even as the Head Master at his school discussed with me his belief that Richard's behavior indicated probable alcohol exposure prior to his birth, I had already begun to suspect such.

Yet despite Richard's impairments, he was able to adjust to hardships that would be difficult even for the most able-minded person to endure. Just a few I would like to mention here…

Richard was extremely young when his mother disappeared from his life, and his memory of her alcoholic-related behaviors was truly heart-wrenching.

There was a period of time when Richard lived in a foster home, separated from his father and his brother, until he could stay with me for a while.

His father died suddenly when he was in middle school, and then his adjustment to a whole new life in my home.

And despite all of this, Richard just kept on going, taking everything in his stride.

I was always tickled at the things that gave him joy, like Frosted Flakes for breakfast, making his own eggs, helping my son work on his car, watching movies with my daughter, playing computer games with my sons, and of course, wrestling with his brother.

Helping others also gave Richard joy. He always offered help to everybody. When it came to helping me clean, or taking in the groceries, putting a piece of furniture together, or just carrying something heavy for me… Richard was always there for me. I don't think there was ever a day that he didn't ask me, "How can I help you, Aunt Sherry?"

Richard's ability to forgive was also remarkable. The word "grudge" was just not in his vocabulary. When he would get angry he just blew off steam, and then he would let it go.

The last thing I'd like to tell you is about the strong love that Richard had for his brother, "Little Bro" he would say. He was always asking about, and worrying about, his brother. Richard was very proud of his younger brother, and in many ways, he looked up to him. When I would watch them together I could see that Richard had the gift of loving, a gift that some might argue is greater than spelling or reading.

Thank you.

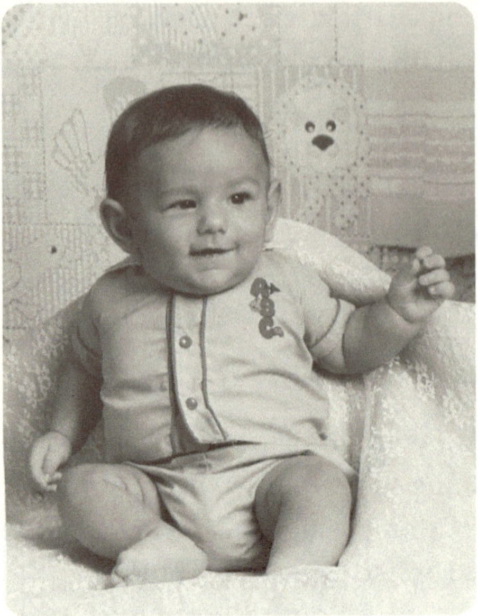

Richard at 8 months

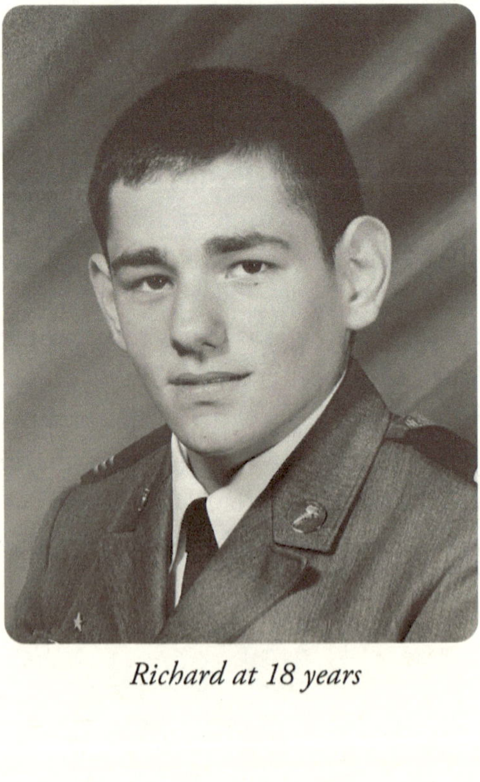

Richard at 18 years

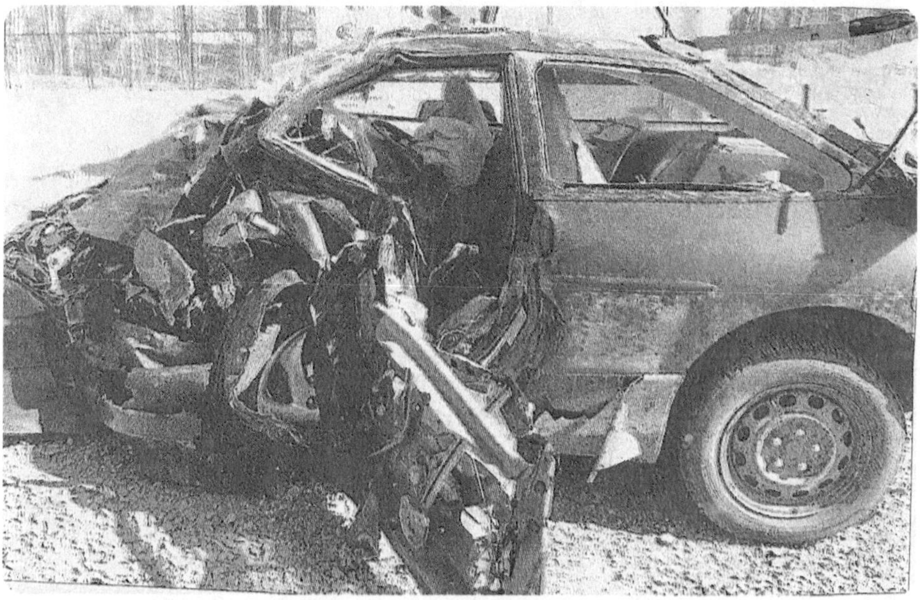

Richard's car after his fatal crash

A 2005 Message to Women from the U.S. Surgeon General:

Advisory on Alcohol Use in Pregnancy

Thirty-two years ago, United States researchers first recognized fetal alcohol syndrome (FAS). FAS is characterized by growth deficiencies (or, decreased growth), abnormal facial features (specific facial features), and central nervous system (or, brain) abnormalities. FAS falls under the spectrum of adverse outcomes caused by prenatal alcohol exposure called Fetal Alcohol Spectrum Disorders (FASD). The discovery of FAS led to considerable public education and awareness initiatives informing women to limit the amount of alcohol they consume while pregnant. But since that time, more has been learned about the effects of alcohol on a fetus. It is now clear that no amount of alcohol can be considered safe.

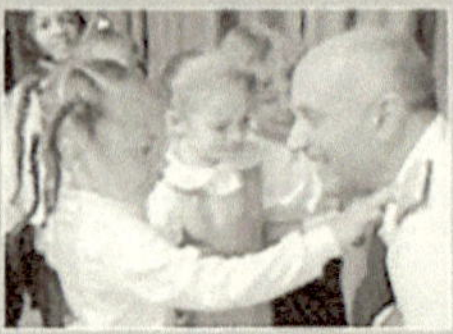

I now wish to emphasize to prospective parents, healthcare practitioners, and all childbearing-aged women, especially those who are pregnant, the importance of not drinking alcohol if a woman is pregnant or considering becoming pregnant.

Based on the current, best science available we now know the following:

- Alcohol consumed during pregnancy increases the risk of alcohol related birth defects, including growth deficiencies, facial abnormalities, central nervous system impairment, behavioral disorders, and impaired intellectual development.
- No amount of alcohol consumption can be considered safe during pregnancy.
- Alcohol can damage a fetus at any stage of pregnancy. Damage can occur in the earliest weeks of pregnancy, even before a woman knows that she is pregnant.
- The cognitive deficits and behavioral problems resulting from prenatal alcohol exposure are lifelong.
- Alcohol-related birth defects are completely preventable.

For these reasons:

1. A pregnant woman should not drink alcohol during pregnancy.
2. A pregnant woman who has already consumed alcohol during her pregnancy should stop in order to minimize further risk.
3. A woman who is considering becoming pregnant should abstain from alcohol.
4. Recognizing that nearly half of all births in the United States are unplanned, women of childbearing age should consult their physician and take steps to reduce the possibility of prenatal alcohol exposure.
5. Health professionals should inquire routinely about alcohol consumption by women of childbearing age, inform them of the risks of alcohol consumption during pregnancy, and advise them not to drink alcoholic beverages during pregnancy.

U.S. Surgeon General,
Vice Admiral Richard H. Carmona, MD, MPH, FACS

Surgeon General's Advisory on Alcohol Use in Pregnancy (front)

For additional information on alcohol use and pregnancy, please visit...

Centers for Disease Control and Prevention (CDC)
www.cdc.gov/ncbddd/fas

National Institute for Alcohol Abuse and Alcoholism (NIAAA)
www.niaaa.nih.gov

Substance Abuse and Mental Health Services Administration (SAMHSA)
Substance Abuse Treatment Facility Locator
www.findtreatment.samhsa.gov

SAMHSA FASD Center for Excellence
www.fascenter.samhsa.gov

National Organization on Fetal Alcohol Syndrome (NOFAS)
www.nofas.org

The Arc of the United States
www.thearc.org

FAS Community Resource Center
www.come-over.to/FASCRC

Fetal Alcohol Syndrome Family Resource Institute (FAS*FRI)
www.fetalalcoholsyndrome.org

FAS Diagnostic & Prevention Network (FAS DPN)
www.depts.washington.edu/fasdpn

Fetal Alcohol and Drug Unit (FADU)
www.depts.washington.edu/fadu

March of Dimes
www.marchofdimes.com

Surgeon General's Advisory on Alcohol Use in Pregnancy (back)

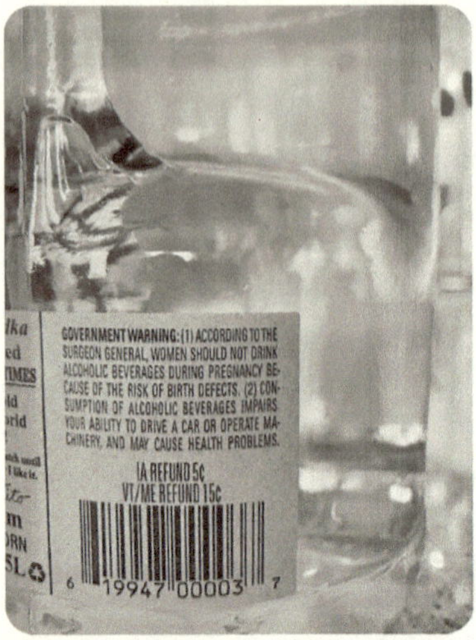

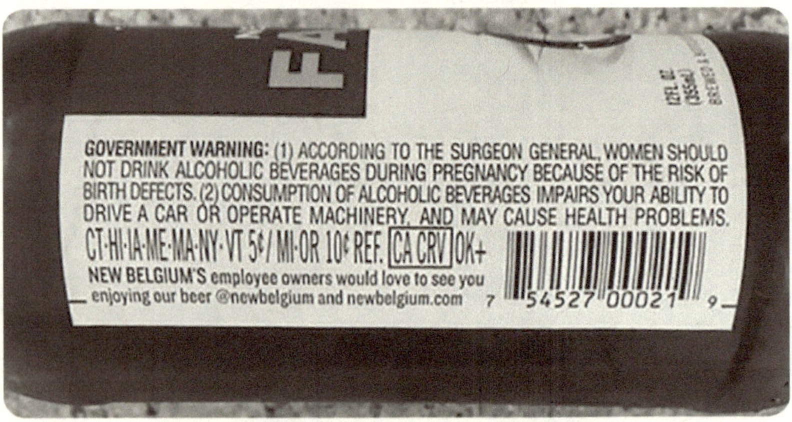

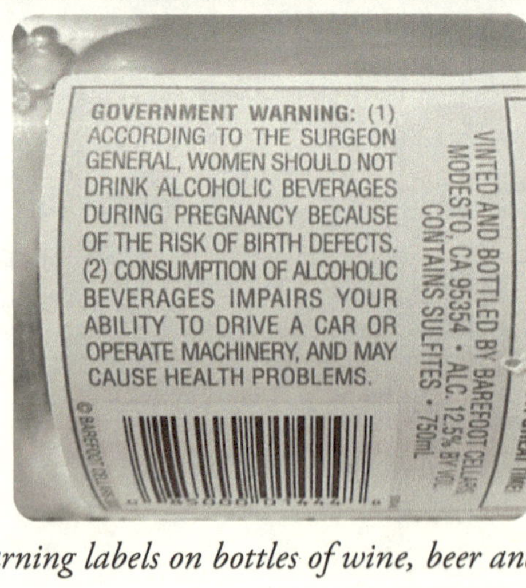

Warning labels on bottles of wine, beer and liquor

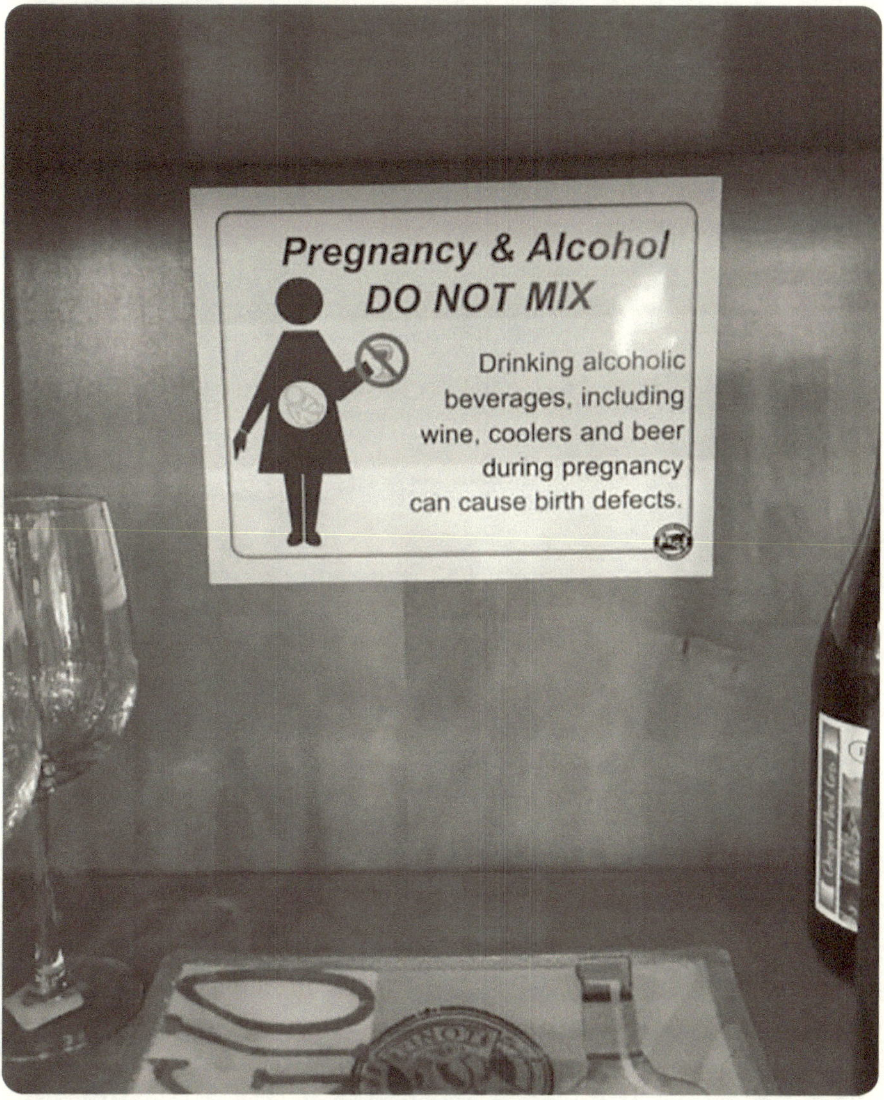
Pregnancy & Alcohol
DO NOT MIX
Drinking alcoholic
beverages, including
wine, coolers and beer
during pregnancy
can cause birth defects.

Warning sign posted in bar

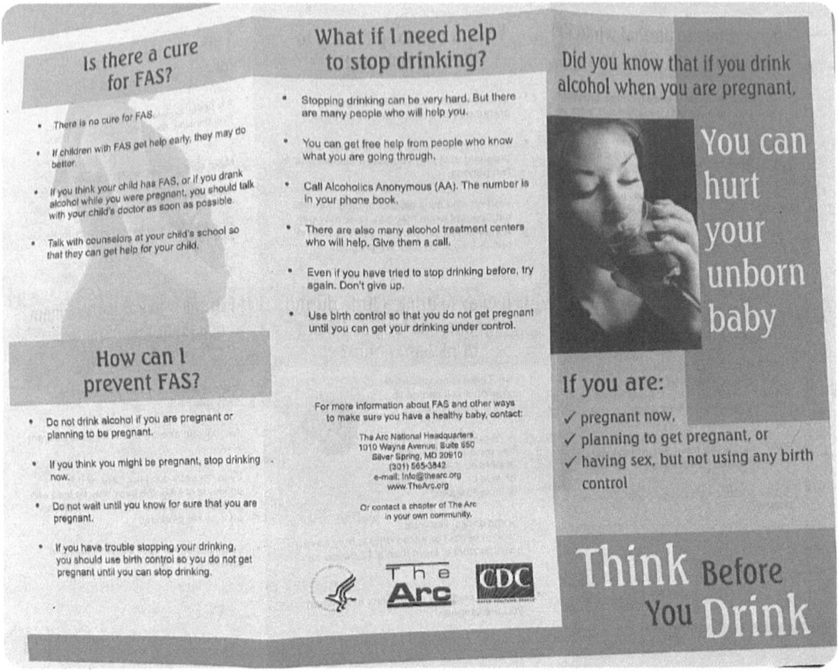

Is there a cure for FAS?

- There is no cure for FAS.
- If children with FAS get help early, they may do better.
- If you think your child has FAS, or if you drank alcohol while you were pregnant, you should talk with your child's doctor as soon as possible.
- Talk with counselors at your child's school so that they can get help for your child.

How can I prevent FAS?

- Do not drink alcohol if you are pregnant or planning to be pregnant.
- If you think you might be pregnant, stop drinking now.
- Do not wait until you know for sure that you are pregnant.
- If you have trouble stopping your drinking, you should use birth control so you do not get pregnant until you can stop drinking.

What if I need help to stop drinking?

- Stopping drinking can be very hard. But there are many people who will help you.
- You can get free help from people who know what you are going through.
- Call Alcoholics Anonymous (AA). The number is in your phone book.
- There are also many alcohol treatment centers who will help. Give them a call.
- Even if you have tried to stop drinking before, try again. Don't give up.
- Use birth control so that you do not get pregnant until you can get your drinking under control.

For more information about FAS and other ways to make sure you have a healthy baby, contact:

The Arc National Headquarters
1010 Wayne Avenue, Suite 650
Silver Spring, MD 20910
(301) 565-3842
e-mail: Info@thearc.org
www.TheArc.org

Or contact a chapter of The Arc in your own community.

Did you know that if you drink alcohol when you are pregnant,

You can hurt your unborn baby

If you are:

✓ pregnant now,
✓ planning to get pregnant, or
✓ having sex, but not using any birth control

Think Before You Drink

CDC FAS Brochure (Front and Back)

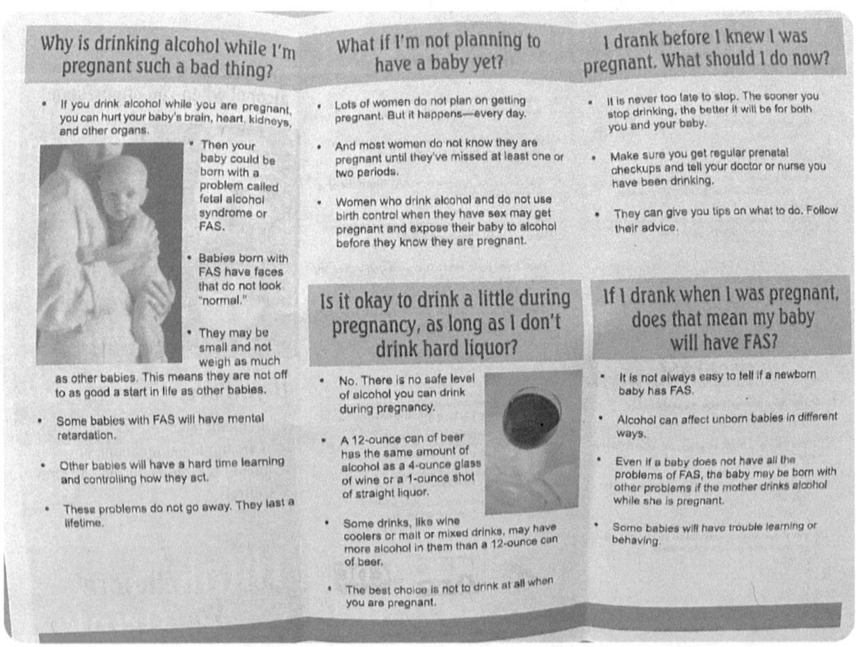

Why is drinking alcohol while I'm pregnant such a bad thing?

- If you drink alcohol while you are pregnant, you can hurt your baby's brain, heart, kidneys, and other organs.
- Then your baby could be born with a problem called fetal alcohol syndrome or FAS.
- Babies born with FAS have faces that do not look "normal."
- They may be small and not weigh as much as other babies. This means they are not off to as good a start in life as other babies.
- Some babies with FAS will have mental retardation.
- Other babies will have a hard time learning and controlling how they act.
- These problems do not go away. They last a lifetime.

What if I'm not planning to have a baby yet?

- Lots of women do not plan on getting pregnant. But it happens—every day.
- And most women do not know they are pregnant until they've missed at least one or two periods.
- Women who drink alcohol and do not use birth control when they have sex may get pregnant and expose their baby to alcohol before they know they are pregnant.

Is it okay to drink a little during pregnancy, as long as I don't drink hard liquor?

- No. There is no safe level of alcohol you can drink during pregnancy.
- A 12-ounce can of beer has the same amount of alcohol as a 4-ounce glass of wine or a 1-ounce shot of straight liquor.
- Some drinks, like wine coolers or malt or mixed drinks, may have more alcohol in them than a 12-ounce can of beer.
- The best choice is not to drink at all when you are pregnant.

I drank before I knew I was pregnant. What should I do now?

- It is never too late to stop. The sooner you stop drinking, the better it will be for both you and your baby.
- Make sure you get regular prenatal checkups and tell your doctor or nurse you have been drinking.
- They can give you tips on what to do. Follow their advice.

If I drank when I was pregnant, does that mean my baby will have FAS?

- It is not always easy to tell if a newborn baby has FAS.
- Alcohol can affect unborn babies in different ways.
- Even if a baby does not have all the problems of FAS, the baby may be born with other problems if the mother drinks alcohol while she is pregnant.
- Some babies will have trouble learning or behaving.

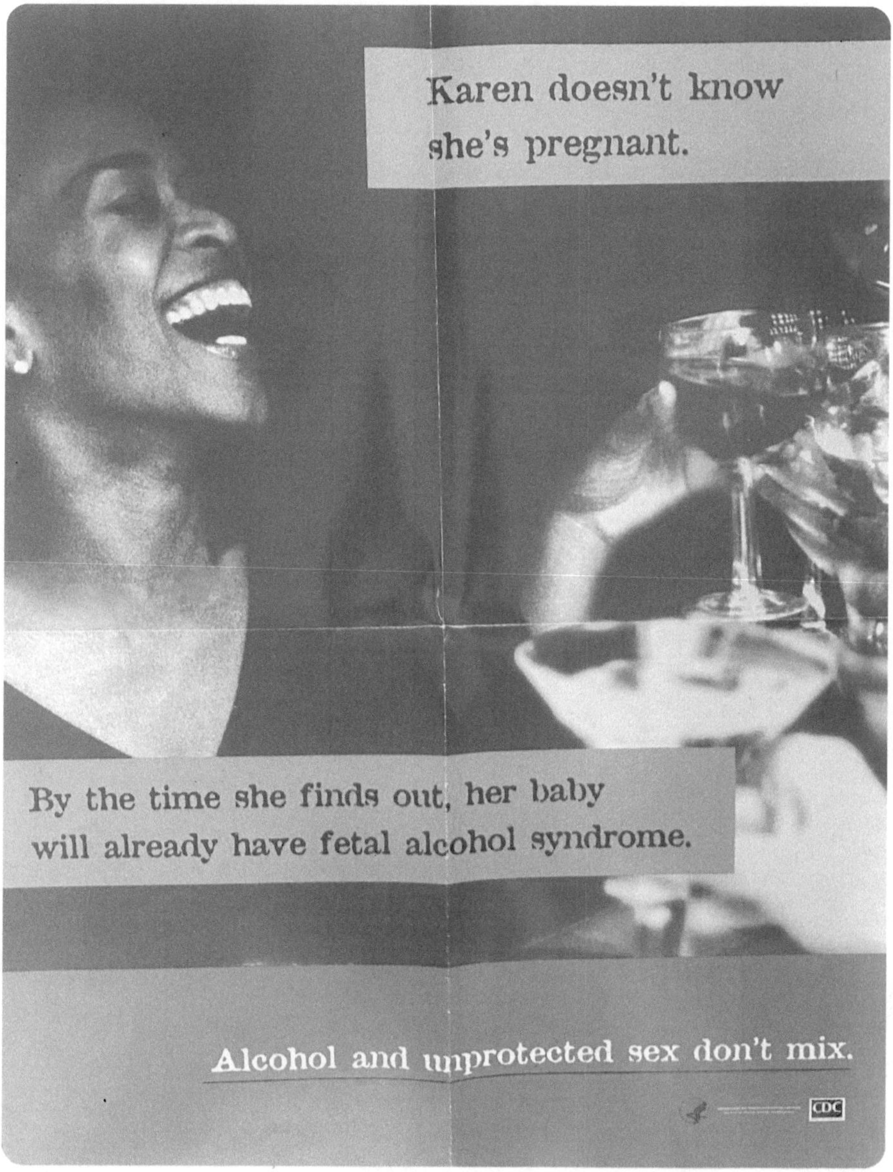

CDC FAS Poster

ABOUT THE AUTHOR

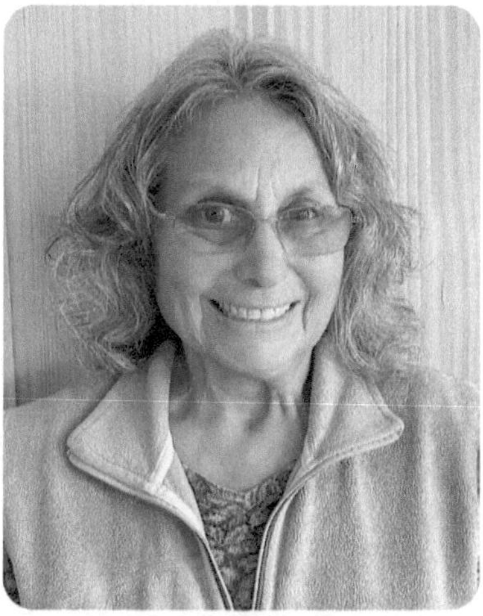

Sherry T. Ford, a graduate of University of Maryland School of Nursing, has been an Advanced Practice Registered Nurse since 1992, with a specialty in Adult Psychiatric and Mental Health Nursing. Her professional career began in Baltimore, Maryland, where she was born and raised.

Initially working as a staff nurse on an inpatient adult behavioral health unit, Sherry later worked as a Certified Nurse Psychotherapist for a substance abuse program, and later as Director of Geropsychiatric Services for a large healthcare system. After moving to Virginia in 2008, she worked in the Quality department for a health insurance company until she retired in 2020.

Sherry has always enjoyed writing and has been published in two nursing journals; Perspectives in Psychiatric Care and RN Magazine. Her hobbies include swimming, hiking, making beaded jewelry, and especially arrowhead hunting- an activity that both her and her husband Tom both delight in.

Sherry and Tom reside in a rural county in the Shenandoah Valley where they both love the beautiful views, their good friends, and visits from their combined children and grandchildren.

www.ingramcontent.com/pod-product-compliance
Lightning Source LLC
LaVergne TN
LVHW101617210926
848480LV00009B/786